LIBRARY OF CONGRESS
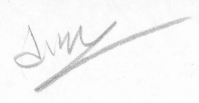

M000238832

Advance praise for *Wisdom Mind: Mindfulness for Cognitively Healthy Older Adults and Those With Subjective Cognitive Decline, Participant Workbook*

"Many of us experience subtle decline in cognitive functioning in the second half of life. While in most this is a sign of normal aging, in some it may progress onward to dementia. However, we know today that we actively support our brain health by mindfulness training. Dr. Smart's manual is an excellent example of how this knowledge from science can serve individual people in maintaining brain function and improving quality of life."

—**Frank Jessen**, MD, University of Cologne

"*Wisdom Mind* is a wonderful tool for clinicians and patients alike! It is based in evidence and specifically designed to support those facing or fearful of cognitive decline. The step-by-step suggestions and practices in the program offer ways to support cognitive wellness as well as cultivate the attitudes of mindfulness that can help all of us face ageing. Thank you Dr. Smart for providing us with a wonderful resource which serves both as intervention and prevention!"

—**Fraser Black**, MD, CCFP(PC), FCFP, Physician/Clinical Professor/Assistant Dean – University of British Columbia, Faculty of Medicine, Art of Living Mindfully (BCALM) Mindfulness Facilitator

"A warmhearted and accessible resource for skillfully meeting the cognitive changes associated with aging. With the practice of mindfulness at its core, *Wisdom Mind* reminds us that along with whatever contractions in mental abilities we may notice, there is also scope for expansion and vibrant cognitive engagement. This book is the perfect guide for learning how to balance the two."

—**Zindel Segal**, PhD, Distinguished Professor of Psychology in Mood Disorders, University of Toronto Scarborough, co-author *The Mindful Way Through Depression*

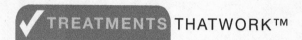 **TREATMENTS** THATWORK™

Editor-In-Chief

David H. Barlow, PhD

Scientific Advisory Board

Anne Marie Albano, PhD

Gillian Butler, PhD

David M. Clark, PhD

Edna B. Foa, PhD

Paul J. Frick, PhD

Jack M. Gorman, MD

Kirk Heilbrun, PhD

Robert J. McMahon, PhD

Peter E. Nathan, PhD

Christine Maguth Nezu, PhD

Matthew K. Nock, PhD

Paul Salkovskis, PhD

Bonnie Spring, PhD

Gail Steketee, PhD

John R. Weisz, PhD

G. Terence Wilson, PhD

Wisdom Mind

Mindfulness for Cognitively Healthy Older Adults and
Those With Subjective Cognitive Decline

PARTICIPANT WORKBOOK

COLETTE M. SMART

With yoga by
KRISTEN SILVEIRA

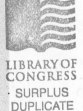

LIBRARY OF
CONGRESS
· SURPLUS
DUPLICATE

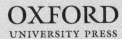

OXFORD
UNIVERSITY PRESS

OXFORD
UNIVERSITY PRESS

Oxford University Press is a department of the University of Oxford. It furthers the University's objective of excellence in research, scholarship, and education by publishing worldwide. Oxford is a registered trade mark of Oxford University Press in the UK and certain other countries.

Published in the United States of America by Oxford University Press
198 Madison Avenue, New York, NY 10016, United States of America.

© Oxford University Press 2021

All rights reserved. No part of this publication may be reproduced, stored in a retrieval system, or transmitted, in any form or by any means, without the prior permission in writing of Oxford University Press, or as expressly permitted by law, by license, or under terms agreed with the appropriate reproduction rights organization. Inquiries concerning reproduction outside the scope of the above should be sent to the Rights Department, Oxford University Press, at the address above.

You must not circulate this work in any other form
and you must impose this same condition on any acquirer.

CIP data is on file at the Library of Congress

ISBN 978–0–19–751012–4

DOI: 10.1093/med/9780197510124.001.0001

9 8 7 6 5 4 3 2 1

Printed by Marquis, Canada

One of the most difficult problems confronting patients with various disorders and diseases is finding the best help available. Everyone is aware of friends or family who have sought treatment from a seemingly reputable practitioner only to find out later from another doctor that the original diagnosis was wrong or the treatments recommended were inappropriate or perhaps even harmful. Most patients, or family members, address this problem by reading everything they can about their symptoms, seeking out information on the internet or aggressively "asking around" to tap knowledge from friends and acquaintances. Governments and health care policymakers are also aware that people in need do not always get the best treatments—something they refer to as *variability in health care practices*.

Now health care systems around the world are attempting to correct this variability by introducing *evidence-based practice*. This simply means that it is in everyone's interest that patients get the most up-to-date and effective care for a particular problem. Health care policymakers have also recognized that it is very useful to give consumers of health care as much information as possible, so that they can make intelligent decisions in a collaborative effort to improve physical health and mental health. This series, Treatments *That Work*™, is designed to accomplish just that. Only the latest and most effective interventions for particular problems are described, in user-friendly language. To be included in this series, each treatment program must pass the highest standards of evidence available, as determined by a scientific advisory board. Thus, when individuals suffering from these problems or their family members seek out an expert clinician who is familiar with these interventions and decides that they are appropriate, patients will have confidence they are receiving the best care available. Of course, only your health care professional can decide on the right mix of treatments for you.

The latest development in evidence-based treatment programs, based on the most up-to-date research and clinical evaluation, is found in unified, transdiagnostic interventions for disorders that share common features and respond to common therapeutic procedures. Deepening understanding of the nature of psychological disorders reveals that many groups of related disorders share important causes and look very similar in terms of behavioral problems and brain function. Thinking of these disorders or problems as related, or on a "spectrum," is the approach now taken by leading therapists and researchers as well as by the authors of the *DSM-5*, the Diagnostic and Statistical Manual of Mental Disorders, 5th Edition. This is because most people with one disorder or problem also have another problem or disorder (referred to as comorbidity). Someone with panic disorder may also have social anxiety as well as depression; these are all emotional disorders. Someone who abuses drugs may also abuse alcohol or cigarettes; these are all addictive disorders. Treatment programs in this series are "unified" because they share a common, unified set of therapeutic procedures that are effective with a whole class of disorders, such as emotional disorders or addictive disorders. Treatment programs are "transdiagnostic" because they are designed to be effective with all of the disorders in that class (emotional or addictive or eating disorders) that somebody might have, rather than just one disorder. Working with one set of therapeutic principles makes it easier and more efficient for you and your therapist and should address all of the problems you may have in a more comprehensive and effective way.

Cognitive aging—or age-related changes in our thinking abilities—is a normal experience in late life, yet it can cause substantial distress. *Wisdom Mind* is an 8-week mindfulness training program specifically designed for cognitively healthy older adults who want to maintain their cognitive abilities at current levels, as well as for older adults who find themselves experiencing some memory loss or other subtle cognitive changes in their thinking abilities that are causing them concern, something we call subjective cognitive decline (SCD).

This mindfulness program is designed to improve cognitive function through the practice of mindfulness as well as to cultivate attitudes of mindfulness as a way to accept the changes and losses in our cognitive abilities that we experience in late life. Explanations are provided in each chapter for why certain techniques or practices are employed. *Wisdom Mind* will be an indispensable resource for older adults interested in using mindfulness to improve their daily lives, and in finding ways to not only navigate the challenges of aging but also to embrace its many gifts.

David H. Barlow, Editor-in-Chief

Treatments *ThatWork*™

Boston, Massachusetts

Contents

Welcome. With great pleasure, I want to take the next few minutes to introduce you to the path on which you will be traveling for the next 8 weeks—the path of mindfulness. My name is Dr. Colette Smart, and I am a clinical neuropsychologist and a psychology professor at the University of Victoria, British Columbia—and the creator of this program.

First of all, I want you to take a moment to congratulate yourself that you are taking this positive step in your life. By engaging fully in this program, you are making a commitment to be kind to yourself and uncover the basic wisdom that already lies in your daily life. You are making a commitment not to avoid or turn away from what is difficult, and instead you are making a decision to turn toward your life and embrace it in its fullness. This is no small effort! As someone who has been practicing and teaching mindfulness for more than 20 years, I take great joy at the idea that other people can benefit from this deeply fulfilling practice. Even though I am not there in person, I look forward to walking this path with you, virtually.

What Is Mindfulness?

You are probably already wondering, "What is mindfulness?" So let me take a moment to talk with you about it. Mindfulness is a contemplative practice that has been around for thousands of years. Although it is practiced within many different spiritual and secular traditions, you do not need to ascribe to any particular belief system to experience the benefits of mindfulness. Our current culture places a lot of emphasis on doing and achieving, and this can cause great distress and suffering for many people as they feel that they have to live up to certain expectations about who they need to be and how they need to perform. In contrast, mindfulness involves learning how to be with your experience as it unfolds moment to moment, without any specific agenda of what your life has to be. Mindfulness is both a set of specific practices and also a particular way of looking at things. It is not a "self-improvement project"; rather, it is a practice of uncovering and discovering a deep sense of curiosity, acceptance, and loving-kindness toward your life as it is, without the need to change or fix things.

Does Mindfulness Actually Work?

Thousands of years of anecdotal evidence suggest that this practice works—otherwise people wouldn't keep doing it! But there is now also systematic scientific research that demonstrates that mindfulness does in fact help many people. The program in which you will be participating is broadly based on the mindfulness-based stress reduction (MBSR) program developed by Dr. Jon Kabat-Zinn at the University of Massachusetts Medical Center. There is now over 30 years' worth of research showing that mindfulness can be helpful with a variety of challenges, including depression, anxiety, chronic pain, psoriasis, and cancer, as well as for individuals simply looking to enhance well-being in their lives. Studies on individuals who practice mindfulness over the long term also suggest positive changes in brain structure and function, including decreased brain shrinkage in old age. For those of you who might be interested, I have included some Further Readings on relevant studies at the end of this Introduction.

How Might This Program Be Helpful to Older Adults?

This particular program, *Wisdom Mind*, is quite special. Back in 2011, I took the standard MBSR program and tailored it specifically for older adults. Instead of wearing a "one-size-fits-all" kind of program, you will be trying on something custom-made just for you. As a clinical neuropsychologist, I have worked for many years in clinical practice with all kinds of people who have struggled with their thinking abilities and emotional well-being, and I know some of the "tricks of the trade" to help people manage these challenges. I have been teaching some form of mindfulness meditation to individuals and groups for more than 15 years. Before developing *Wisdom Mind*, I was the co-investigator of a 2-year study looking at the benefits of mindfulness training in people with traumatic brain injury, which gave me some ideas about how to tailor mindfulness to different people experiencing challenges in their thinking abilities. This knowledge was combined with my experiences as a human being on this path of meditation, with a deep appreciation for its capacity to bring kindness and appreciation to my life.

Much of my formal clinical training and work as a psychologist has involved older adults, and I understand the concerns that often come up about changes in mental and emotional functions as we age. Our minds may slow down, we may have trouble coming up with the right word, we may feel less sharp than we used to. Many of these changes are part and parcel of getting older. In today's fast-paced world of technology and endless information overload, these natural changes in our state of mind can be a source of great distress and worry, which often makes it even harder to think clearly. Unfortunately, our society tends not to embrace aging as something positive and meaningful. That said, research suggests that one thing really does seem to improve as we age: our sense of wisdom. Wisdom involves being able to take a step back, see the big picture, and appreciate the value in our experience whether it feels pleasurable or challenging. Wisdom does not depend on being smart or intelligent; it is about being open to our experience and learning from life's lessons with an open heart and mind. It involves tuning in to our own emotional life and, in doing so, connecting more deeply with the emotional life and struggles of those around us.

Cultivating wisdom is very much supported by mindfulness practice. I like the idea of focusing on wisdom for older adults because it involves capitalizing on something you might already be good at. This is why I developed this program called *Wisdom Mind*. Research studies conducted on this program indicate that participants experience improvements in their mood, their perceived memory abilities (memory self-efficacy), cognitive measures such as attention, and also positive changes in brain structure and function. Those studies are included in the Further Readings section at the end of this Introduction. As a result of this research, I am now very grateful to be able to bring this program to you.

The final thing I want to discuss with you is how best to approach this program. The amount of benefit you get from this program depends very much on how much you put into it. Mindfulness training has been demonstrated many times over to significantly impact mental and emotional well-being, but only if you do the practices regularly. You will be coming to a weekly group, but you will be doing most of the work on your own, outside of the group, in your between-group practices. It is common for people to encounter challenges in making time to implement these practices, but the group is here to support you in these challenges and help you to find ways to incorporate the practices into your daily life.

Back to the specific "tailoring" for older adults: Your group facilitator will make some specific suggestions about how to implement these practices in your daily life. These include:

1. **Repetition**—Sometimes things might seem repetitive, like a broken record. But the more repetition we get, the more things are likely to stick.
2. **Multiple modalities**—Sometimes that repetition will come in the form of reading the material, hearing it on a downloadable audio recording, and listening to your group facilitator discuss it in the session. Learning things in different contexts can increase the chances you will remember it better later on.
3. **Prospective memory**—Prospective memory consists of being able to remember to do things in the future, like brush your teeth, take your medication, or remember your doctor's appointment. This also includes remembering when it is time to practice mindfulness! Sometimes it gets harder to use prospective memory as we get older (or, if you're like me, it has been a lifelong struggle!). Each week, the group facilitator will discuss explicitly how you can cue yourself to remember to do your mindfulness practice so that you have the best chance of benefiting from the program.

I mentioned before that this program is about learning how to *be* rather than *do*, but paradoxically we actually have to practice learning how to be. However, rather than feeling as if this is another thing to add to your "to-do" list, I invite you to approach these practices as a way to uncover your life. You may have heard the expression "practice makes perfect." To me, this emphasizes getting it right or being good. Instead, I would like you think about it this way: "practice is perfection." This means that the most important thing is to give it a try—that's what really counts. And by giving something a try, you realize the perfection that has been waiting for you in your life all along.

Finally, as noted earlier, *Wisdom Mind* is broadly based on Dr. Kabat-Zinn's MBSR program, but it contains enough unique elements for it to be a standalone program. That said, Kabat-Zinn's 1990 book *Full Catastrophe Living* may be a great optional resource for you during this program. That book describes the MBSR program and provides a highly accessible resource in terms of understanding what mindfulness is and how we can cultivate it in daily life. In each chapter of this *Workbook*, a reference is made to supplemental chapters from this Kabat-Zinn book in case you are interested in reviewing those chapters as a supplemental support.

Suggested Readings

Azulay, J., Smart, C. M., Mott, T., & Cicerone, K. D. (2013). A pilot study examining the effects of mindfulness-based stress reduction on symptoms of chronic mild traumatic brain injury/post-concussive syndrome. *Journal of Head Trauma Rehabilitation, 28*, 323–331.

Baer, R. A. (2003). Mindfulness training as a clinical intervention: A conceptual and empirical review. *Clinical Psychology: Science and Practice, 10*, 125–143.

Fox, K. C., Dixon, M. L., Nijeboer, S., Girn, M., Floman, J. L., Lifshitz, M., Ellamil, M., Sedlmeier, P., & Christoff, K. (2016). Functional neuroanatomy of meditation: A review and meta-analysis of 78 functional neuroimaging investigations. *Neuroscience and Biobehavioral Reviews, 65*, 208–228.

Fox, K. C., Nijeboer, S., Dixon, M. L., Floman, J. L., Ellamil, M., Rumak, S. P., Sedlmeier, P., & Christoff, K. (2014). Is meditation associated with altered brain structure? A systematic review and meta-analysis of morphometric neuroimaging in meditation practitioners. *Neuroscience and Biobehavioral Reviews, 43*, 48–73.

Holzel, B. K., Carmody, J., Vangel, M., Congleton, C., Yerramsetti, S. M., Gard, T., & Lazar, S. W. (2011). Mindfulness practice leads to increases in regional brain gray matter density. *Psychiatry Research: Neuroimaging, 191*, 36–43.

Kabat-Zinn, J. (1990). *Full catastrophe living: Using the wisdom of your body and mind to face stress, pain, and illness* (rev. ed.). Bantam.

Lazar, S. W., Kerr, C. E., Wasserman, R. H., Gray, J. R., Greve, D. N., Treadway M. T., McGarvey, M., Quinn, B. T., Dusek, J. A., Benson, H., Rauch, S. L., Moore, C. I., & Fischl, B. (2005). Meditation experience is associated with cortical thickness. *Neuroreport, 16*, 1893–1897.

Lutz, A., Slagter, H. A., Dunne, J. D., & Davidson, R. J. (2008). Attention regulation and monitoring in meditation. *Trends in Cognitive Sciences, 12*, 163–169.

MacLean, K. A., Ferrer, E., Aichele, S. R., Bridwell, D. A., Zanesco, A. P., Jacobs, T. L., King, B. G., Rosenberg, E. L., Sahdra, B. K., Shaver, P. R., Wallace, B. A., Mangun, G. R., & Saron, C. D. (2010). Intensive meditation training improves perceptual discrimination and sustained attention. *Psychological Science, 21,* 829–839.

Sedlmeier, P., Eberth, J., Schwarz, M., Zimmermann, D., Haarig, F., Jaeger, S., & Kunze, S. (2012). The psychological effects of meditation: A meta-analysis. *Psychological Bulletin, 138,* 1139–1171. doi: 10.1037/a0028168

Smart, C. M., & Segalowitz, S. J. (2017). Respond, don't react: The influence of mindfulness training on performance monitoring in older adults. *Cognitive, Affective, and Behavioral Neuroscience, 17,* 1151–1163. doi: 10.3758/s13415-017-0539-3

Smart, C. M., Segalowitz, S. J., Mulligan, B. P., Koudys, J., & Gawryluk, J. (2016). Mindfulness training for older adults with subjective cognitive decline: Results from a pilot randomized controlled trial. *Journal of Alzheimer's Disease, 52,* 757–774.

CHAPTER 1

Use this space to take notes from today's session—including the "take-home points."

Foundations of Mindfulness—Attitudes and Commitment

In this program, we are going to be learning different practices to cultivate the experience of the present moment. These practices will be our vehicle for the journey. But without a roadmap, it does not matter whether we have a Mercedes-Benz or a tractor-trailer—we are quickly going to get lost. As we embark on the journey, it can be helpful to review and think about the *attitudes of mindfulness* as our roadmap:

1. **Non-judging**: Mindfulness is about cultivating a stance of an impartial observer or witness to our experience. To do this, we have to start becoming aware of our tendency to judge and categorize everything as good or bad, pleasurable or painful, and so on. Other things we are completely indifferent to. Most of these judgments have little objective basis, yet they have the potential to cause great suffering.

2. **Patience**: In our current cultural climate in the West, there is a heavy emphasis on doing and achieving, which leads to irritability and impatience when things don't happen on our time-line. Instead, in this program, we learn to cultivate patience, which is a form of wisdom— being willing to trust that situations will unfold according to the timeline that they need, not what we impose on them.

3. **Beginner's mind**: All too often we let our habitual thinking tell us we "know" how a situation is—we've been there, done that, and don't need to bother investing any time or energy getting to know it any further. In this program, we bring a beginner's mind to both formal and in-formal practices, and then we can experience moments of our life—what once seemed routine and monotonous—as fresh and alive.

4. **Trust**: Developing basic trust in ourselves and our experience is integral to mindfulness training. We might be used to putting our trust in other people, such as a partner, loved ones, powerful politicians, and so on. Instead, in this practice we learn to trust ourselves and in doing so take responsibility for the course of our own lives.

5. **Non-striving**: In this program you will see the tendency to judge your meditation as good or bad, and question whether and how much you are making progress. This goal-oriented mindset runs counter to mindfulness, which is about giving up the need to get it right and be good, and instead is about learning to work with what you have.

6. **Acceptance**: Much of why we suffer is because we reject or resist our experience—it's not what we want or what we signed up for. Acceptance means seeing things clearly as they are. This does not mean passive resignation—it means we acknowledge the current situation for what it is, and take this as the working basis for the next step in our life.

7. **Letting go**: Attachment to pleasure and aversion to pain dominate many of our lives. In learning to let go, we give up that attachment and let the situation unfold as it needs to.

As part of your between-session practice, you may be asked to listen to one or more audio files. These files may be given to you by your program facilitator, or you can download them from the Treatments That Work website at www. oxfordclinicalpsych.com/WisdomMind.

The object of mindfulness practice is not to "be good" or "get it right." That said, the more you try the between-session exercises, the more likely you are to truly benefit from this program. When you are having difficulties making the practices happen, remember to be kind to yourself and do not let "beating yourself up" become an obstacle to trying.

Your between-session practices for this week are:

1. (Optional) Read Chapter 1 from *Full Catastrophe Living* ("Moments to Live").
2. Practice the Body Scan for 6 days.
3. Complete "For the Participant 1.3A: Nine Dots Exercise."
4. Listen to the audio titled "Mindful Eating" to give you guidance on this activity, and then eat at least one or two meals mindfully over the coming week.
5. Notice where you go on auto-pilot.

Learning a new skill means practice, and finding a regular time will help. Write down three different times that you think might be good times to practice the Body Scan this week:

Three times I might practice this week are:

1.
2.
3.

How will you remember to practice? Some examples might be programming your watch or your phone with an alarm, or pairing it with a regularly occurring event such as brushing your teeth before bed. Write down some possible strategies:

1.
2.
3.

For next week: Remember to bring this *Workbook*, a mat/blanket, and your planner.

Body Scan Practice Log

Please make a note here of when you practiced, for how long you practiced, what you noticed when you practiced, and if there were any obstacles to practicing if you did not do it on a particular day.

Day/time of practice	What did you notice (e.g., thoughts, feelings, sensations)?	What obstacles did you notice getting in the way of doing the practice?

Nine Dots Exercise and Mindful Eating

A: Nine Dots Exercise

Connect all of these dots with only four straight lines, without lifting your pen/pencil, and without retracing over any of the lines.

B: Mindful Eating

Jot down some notes about your Mindful Eating experience here:

Use this space to take notes from today's session—including the "take-home points."

As part of your between-session practice, you may be asked to listen to one or more audio files. These files may be given to you by your program facilitator, or you can download them from the Treatments That Work website at www. oxfordclinicalpsych.com/WisdomMind.

This week we will use the Body Scan to continue to develop our ability to connect with our present experience. The body is very concrete, which is often why people find it more accessible when they start out with mindfulness practice. We will also add the first short Sitting Practice. It might help if you try the sitting practice right after you do the Body Scan. Not only will this give you one less thing you need to remember, but doing the Body Scan first might make the Sitting Practice a little easier, too. We will also continue trying to find "moments of mindfulness" in daily life using the assigned homework practices.

Your between-session practices for this week are:

1. Practice the Body Scan for 6 days.
2. Do the 10-minute Sitting Practice for 6 days.
3. Listen to the audio titled "Ordinary Magic" to give you guidance on this activity, and then pick one routine activity to do mindfully.
4. Start noticing slip-ups.

Again, it is important to note that the more you practice, the more benefit you will likely get out of it. Last week you got to experiment with some different times to practice. This week, try to select one regular time to practice and commit to that time.

My time to practice this week will be:

_____

How are you going to remember to practice this week? Write down what strategy you will use to make sure you know it's time to practice:

_____

_____

For next week: Remember to bring your *Workbook*, a mat/blanket to do Mindful Yoga in class, and your planner/calendar. Please dress comfortably.

Tracking Cognitive Slip-Ups

It is common for people of all ages to have slips in their thinking. Maybe we have problems coming up with the right word or putting a name to a face, or we find that things just take longer than they used to. One of the reasons people have slips is because they are distracted and their minds are wandering, thinking about something else. In other words, they are on auto-pilot.

Over the next week, jot down some notes about times you have slipped up. Where was your mind when it happened—were you mind-wandering, or were you in the present moment?

What was the slip-up?	Were you present when it occurred, or were you on auto-pilot?

Body Scan Practice Log

Please make a note here of when you practiced, for how long you practiced, what you noticed when you practiced, and if there were any obstacles to practicing if you did not do it on a particular day.

Day/time of practice	What did you notice (e.g., thoughts, feelings, sensations)?	What obstacles did you notice getting in the way of doing the practice?

FOR THE PARTICIPANT 2.3

Short Sitting (Focused Attention) Practice

Basic Sitting Practice, or "mindfulness of breathing," is the foundation practice in this program. As Jon Kabat-Zinn says in the title of one of his books, "wherever you go, there you are"—meaning that if we can learn to attend to something as simple as our breath, we can come back to the present moment any place and any time because our breath is always with us. This week we will start small. Remember that "practice is perfection" and that the most important thing is that you give it a try and you do it regularly. Resist the temptation to judge it as a "good" or "bad" experience.

Day/time of practice	What was the practice like for you?

Mindful Routine Activity ("Ordinary Magic")

Pick one routine activity (e.g., washing dishes, taking a shower, emptying the garbage) and commit to trying it mindfully. Pick something that is simple and doable. You may find it easier if you try it right after one of the formal practices (i.e., Body Scan or Sitting Practice). Jot down some notes about your experience.

Did You Know?

Mentally and physically stimulating activities add to our cognitive reserve—our mental bank account that can help reduce our risk for cognitive decline.

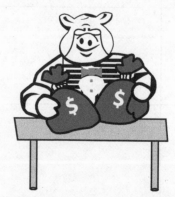

Use this space to take notes from today's session—including the "take-home points."

As part of your between-session practice, you may be asked to listen to one or more audio files. These files may be given to you by your program facilitator, or you can download them from the Treatments That Work website at www. oxfordclinicalpsych.com/WisdomMind.

Mindfulness is not about "being a good meditator." It's about using the formal and informal practices to learn how to come back to our present experience, so that we can actually do it—live it—in our daily life. The practices this week are helping us transition more into "meditation in daily life." This includes increasing the length of our sitting practice, letting go of the Body Scan, and now trying a mindful movement practice (i.e., yoga), as well as capturing pleasant events as they happen throughout our week. We will also notice times where we have a mental slip, and when this causes a strong emotional reaction ("slips and falls").

Your between-session practices for this week are:

1. (Optional) Read Chapter 6 from *Full Catastrophe Living* ("Yoga *Is* Meditation").
2. Practice Mindful Yoga I for 6 days (and fill out the practice log).
3. Do the 20-minute Sitting Practice (Focused Attention) for 6 days (and fill out the practice log).
4. Fill out your Pleasant Events Tracking Log.
5. Start noticing your slips and falls (listen to audio and track them in your log).

Again, it is important to note that the more you practice, the more benefit you will likely get out of it. Last week you got to experiment with some different times to practice. This week, try to select one regular time to practice and commit to that time.

My time to practice this week will be:

_____

How are you going to remember to practice this week? Write down what strategy you will use to make sure you know it's time to practice:

_____

_____

For next week: Remember to bring your *Workbook*, a mat/blanket to do Mindful Yoga II in class, and your planner/calendar. Please dress comfortably.

Sitting Practice Log (Focused Attention, 20 Minutes)

Even though sitting for longer may seem challenging, many people often find that, in sitting longer, they can actually experience the thoughts in their mind settle down. We start to experience a "breath of fresh air" between the thoughts.

You might find yourself inclined to judge your practice—"Am I doing it right? This is boring. I'm so tired." And on and on. Regard any comments to yourself just the same as any other thoughts—without trying to change them, ignore them, or actively suppress them—and simply acknowledge that they are there and let them pass by. This should be done with a light touch, like a feather touching a bubble. Remember, "practice is perfection."

Day/time of practice	What was the practice like for you?

The Attention Hierarchy

Attention is the **most fundamental cognitive process in the brain**. It is the foundation on which all of our other cognitive abilities are built. Attention problems are common in the majority of neurological disorders, and even psychological difficulties such as depression and anxiety. Attention is a complex process that involves many different facets that each build on one another, as shown on this diagram:

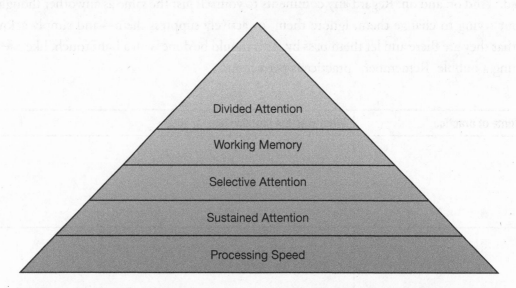

Processing speed refers to how fast we are able to complete a task. In today's busy world, and also in Western culture, there is often an emphasis on speed, which can place extra pressure on us if we have attention difficulties.

Sustained attention is the ability to focus on one thing for an extended period of time. An example might be reading a book or watching a television show.

Selective attention refers to our ability to keep our attention on something when there are distractions, such as reading at a coffee shop or following a conversation at a large social gathering.

Working memory refers to our ability to keep information in mind and manipulate that information, if needed. Examples include trying to figure out how to make change (i.e., mental arithmetic) and trying to remember the confirmation number given to you over the phone by a customer service representative.

Divided attention refers to our ability to keep track of two things at the same time, such as taking notes while someone is talking in a meeting.

Aside from having a neurological and/or psychological disorder, there are many things that can affect our ability to pay attention on a day-to-day basis, such as:

- Extreme stress
- Sleep and fatigue
- Caffeine levels and other medications that affect the brain
- Blood sugar levels
- Motivation (e.g., boredom)
- Impact of normal aging on the brain

The impact of attention problems can be widespread. We might be more prone to making silly mistakes (i.e., cognitive slip-ups), or missing important details in conversation, or having difficulty doing things efficiently. We might also have more difficulty regulating our emotions.

Do you have a sense of where you are having problems with attention?

_____

_____

The good news is, attention can be trained and get better with consistent practice, including the practice of mindfulness! In this program, we will be actively training our ability to pay attention in a mindful way. When we do practices such as Focused Attention, we are starting at the bottom of the hierarchy, working on our sustained and selective attention. As we become more proficient with this, we start moving up the hierarchy toward divided attention—this is when we work on the practices of Open Monitoring and Loving-Kindness, coming later in the program.

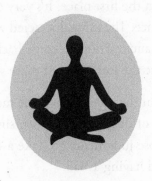

Introducing Slips and Falls

It is common for people of all ages to have slips in their thinking. Maybe we have problems coming up with the right word, putting a name to a face, or finding that things just take longer than they used to.

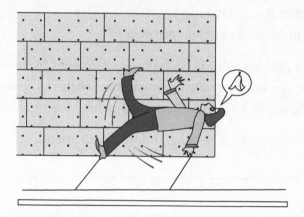

As we get older, these slips happen more often. They might get in the way of our routine activities, such as conversations or grocery shopping. At times we might notice a slip and then get very upset by it or have negative thoughts like "What is wrong with me? Why can't I do this? I must be losing my mind!" When these negative thoughts start cranking up, it can make it even harder to think clearly and focus on what we need to do, compounding the problem and making it worse. It knocks us down. We can think of having a negative response to the slip as a "fall."

How can mindfulness practice help? The practices you will be learning can help us focus our state of mind so we have fewer slip-ups in the first place. It's very common for people these days to be thinking of many, many things at once. The more distracted we are, the more likely we are to have slip-ups. So practicing mindfulness and learning to come back to the present moment and attend to what we are doing might decrease the frequency of these slip-ups in the first place.

But as described earlier, it's a fact that the older we get, the more prone we are to slip-ups. So why beat ourselves up about it? Instead of doing that, we can simply acknowledge with kindness to ourselves that we had a slip, let those judgments go, take a deep breath, and come back to this moment. Then we can at least avoid having a "fall."

Slips and Falls Tracking Log

Over the next week, jot down some places where you had a slip-up, and then whether you had a "fall" over it. You are not trying to change or do anything different right now. The first step is just to get to know yourself and learn how your particular mind operates.

What was the slip-up?	Did you have a "fall" (i.e., negative emotions or judgments about the original slip)?

Mindful Yoga I Practice Log

Please make a note here of when you practiced, for how long you practiced, what you noticed when you practiced, and if there were any obstacles to practicing if you did not do it on a particular day.

Day/time of practice	What did you notice (e.g., thoughts, feelings, sensations)?	What obstacles did you notice getting in the way of doing the practice?

FOR THE PARTICIPANT 3.6

Mindful Yoga I—Demonstration of the Postures

Below are some photographs demonstrating what the postures look like. Remember, it's less important how the pose looks, and more important that you approach the poses mindfully and to the best of your ability.

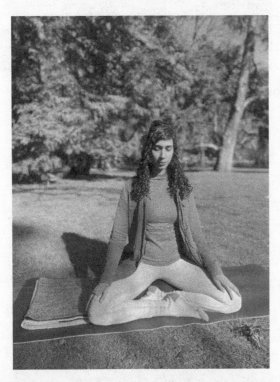
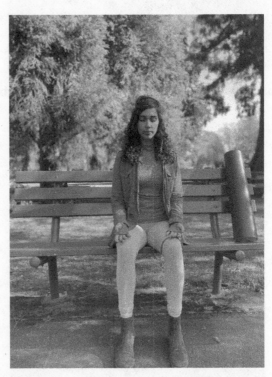

Posture 1: Sitting (either on the floor, or on a chair)

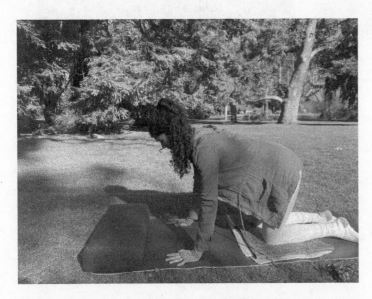

Posture 2: Table Top Position (on the floor; if seated, one can visualize this movement)

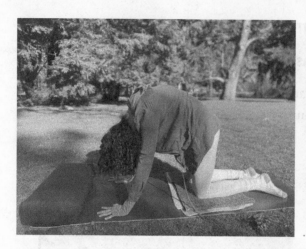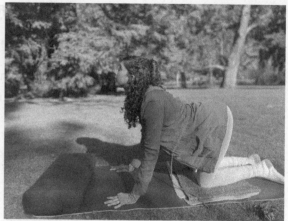

Postures 3 and 4: Cat and Cow (on the floor, above, and on a chair, below)

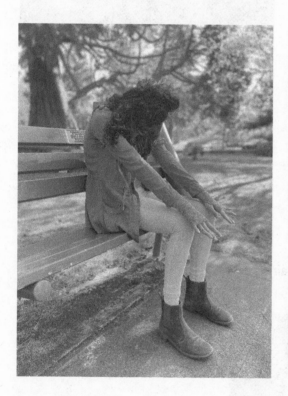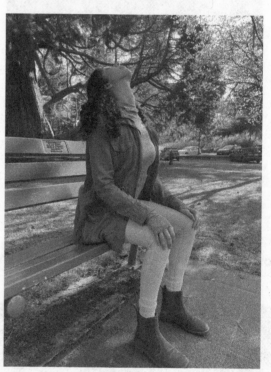

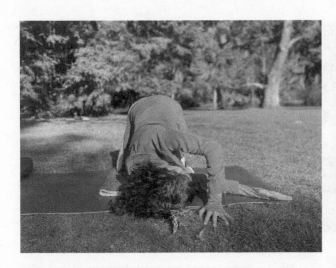

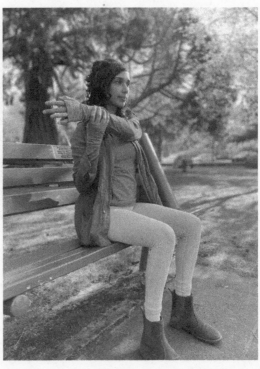

Posture 5: Shoulder Stretch (on the floor and in a chair)

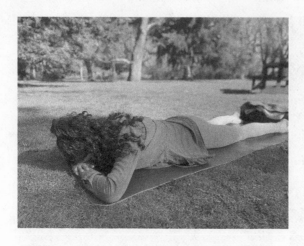 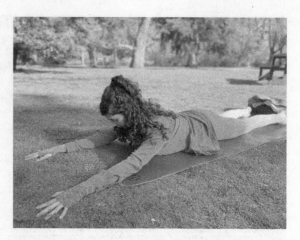

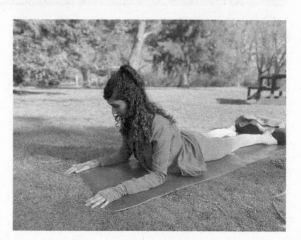

Posture 6: Back Bend (on the floor) — flat, "Superman", and "Sphinx" options

30

Posture 7: Coming Out of Back Bend (on the floor)

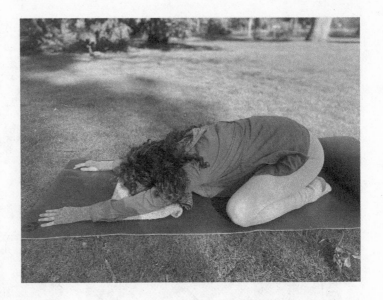

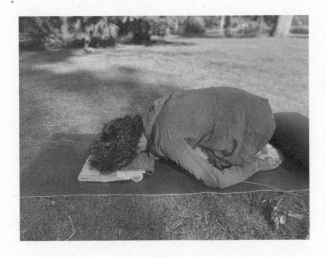

Posture 8: Child's Pose (on the floor) or Forward Fold (on a chair)

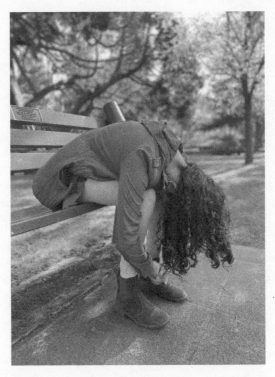

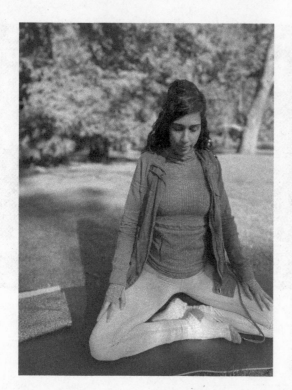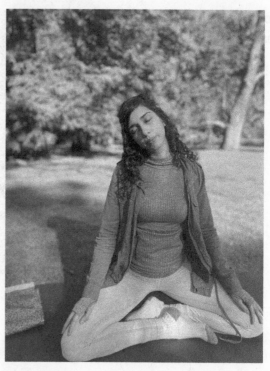

Posture 9: Shoulder and Neck Stretches (on the floor or seated)

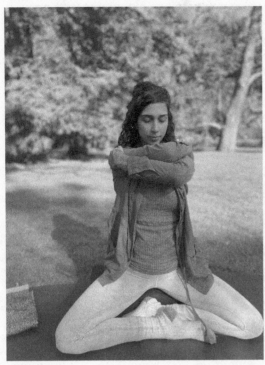

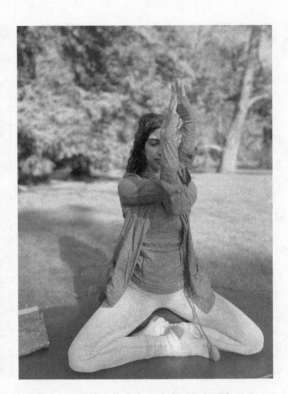

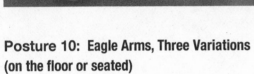

Posture 10: Eagle Arms, Three Variations (on the floor or seated)

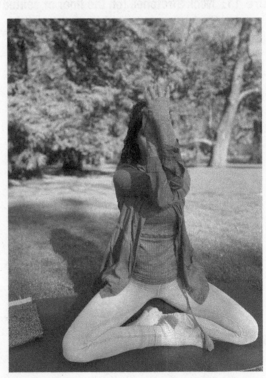

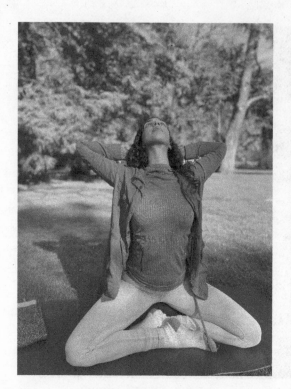 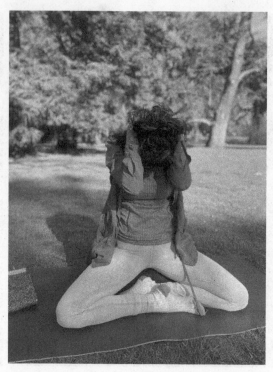

Posture 11: Neck Stretches (on the floor or seated)

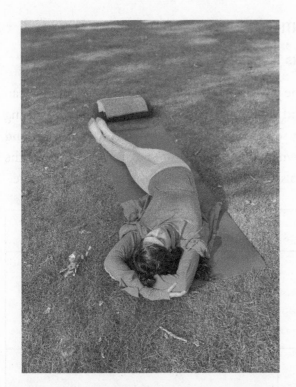

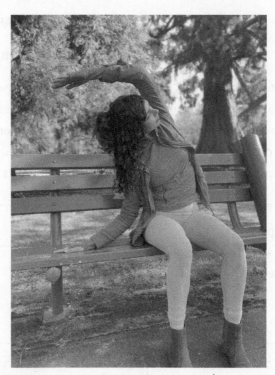

Posture 12: Side Body Stretch (on the floor and in a chair)

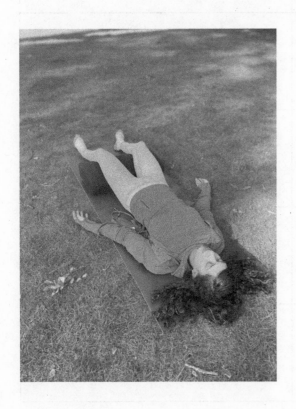

Posture 13: *Svasana* (lying down; can be adapted for the chair)

Did You Know?

Just thinking about a certain type of body movement activates many of the same brain areas as when you actually make that movement. If you find yourself having physical challenges with the yoga postures, try visualizing yourself making the movement instead. Your brain might not know the difference!

35

Pleasant Events Tracking Log

For the next week, set the intention to capture one pleasant moment each day. This does not mean you have to purposefully set up some grand and exciting activity to do. It could be capturing something simple like hearing a child's laughter, seeing a leaf falling off a tree, or sharing a kind word with a loved one. The closer you can jot down your observations to the time of the event, the better you will likely remember it. But you can also reflect at the end of the day, too; that's fine.

Day	What was the pleasant event?	What thoughts, feelings, and sensations did you observe during the experience?

CHAPTER 4

Session 4: Paying Attention to the Commentator

Use this space to take notes from today's session—including the "take-home points."

As part of your between-session practice, you may be asked to listen to one or more audio files. These files may be given to you by your program facilitator, or you can download them from the Treatments That Work website at www. oxfordclinicalpsych.com/WisdomMind.

This week we will continue trying to build a bridge from the formal practice to our daily life. We will continue with Sitting Practice as the foundation, and move into a second sequence of yoga. By recording your pleasant events and slips and falls last week, you may have started to become aware of something called the "commentator"—the voice that is always making judgments about everything that is happening in your experience. This week you will start tracking unpleasant events and, alongside this, start making note of what your commentator is like: Is it silly, angry, anxious, sad, entitled, "disengaged"? What do you notice? For now, simply notice and become familiar.

Your between-session practices for this week are:

1. (Optional) Read Chapter 24 from *Full Catastrophe Living* ("Working With Emotional Pain").
2. Practice Mindful Yoga II for 6 days (and fill out the practice log).
3. Do the 20-minute sitting practice ("Focused Attention") for 6 days (and fill out the practice log).
4. Fill out your Unpleasant Events Tracking Log.
5. Start paying attention to the commentator.

This week, try to select one regular time to practice and commit to that time.

My time to practice this week will be:

_____

How are you going to remember to practice this week? Write down what strategy you will use to make sure you know it's time to practice:

_____

_____

For next week: Remember to bring your *Workbook*, a mat/blanket, and your planner/calendar.

Sitting Practice Log (Focused Attention, 20 Minutes)

Continue your Sitting Practice this week. Be kind to yourself with the practice. Remember, the practice is not just about being continuously focused on the breath, or about "not thinking." Rather, try to observe the dance that occurs between moments when you are on the breath and moments when you have departed. The moment you realize you are gone is the chance you are given to come back.

Day/time of practice	What was the practice like for you?

The **"Commentator"**: Pay attention to the character that sits on your shoulder and comments about what you think, feel, say, and do. Without trying to change it, what do you notice?

Mindful Yoga II Practice Log

Please make a note here of when you practiced, for how long you practiced, what you noticed when you practiced, and if there were any obstacles to practicing if you did not do it on a particular day.

Day/time of practice	What did you notice (e.g., thoughts, feelings, sensations)?	What obstacles did you notice getting in the way of doing the practice?

Mindful Yoga II—Demonstration of the Postures

Below are some photographs demonstrating what the postures look like. Remember, it's less important how the pose looks and more important that you approach the poses mindfully and to the best of your ability.

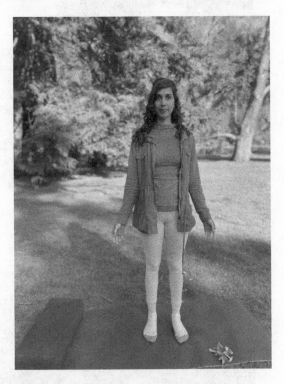 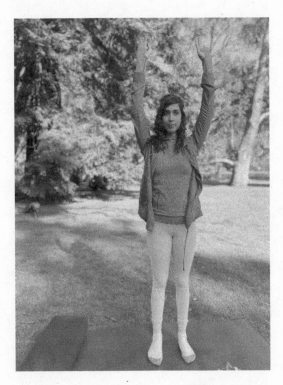

Posture 1: Mountain Pose (standing)

Posture 2: Forward Fold

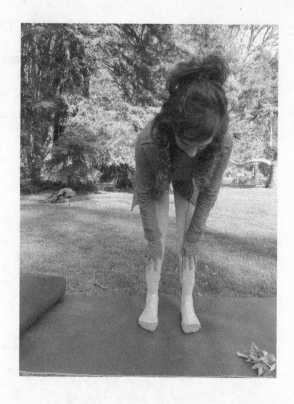

Posture 3: Warrior I

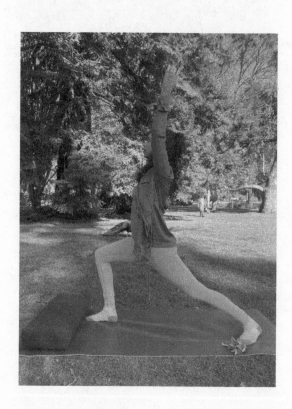

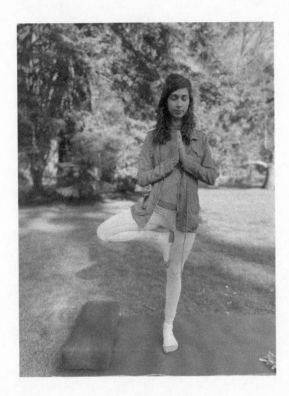

Posture 4: Balancing Tree Posture

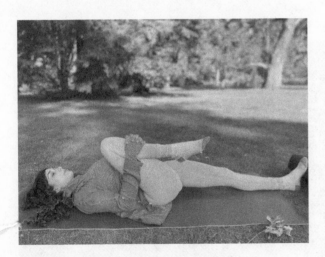

**Posture 5: Knee-to-Chest Pose
(on the floor and on a chair)**

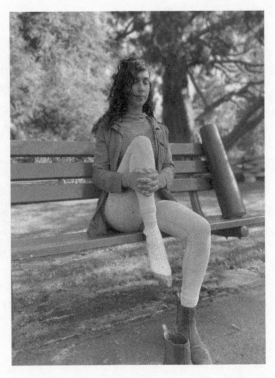

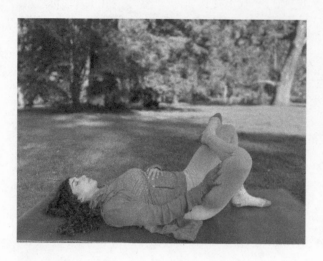

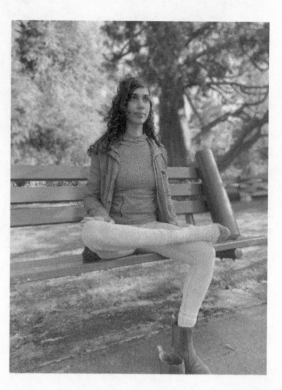

Posture 6: Figure-Four (on the floor and on a chair)

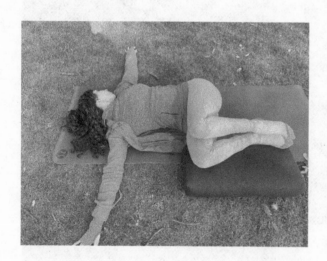

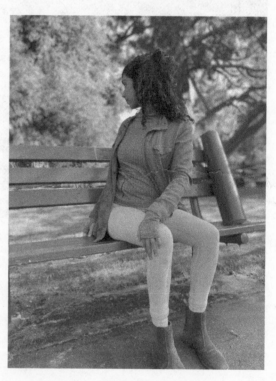

Posture 7: Twist (on the floor and on a chair)

Unpleasant Events Tracking Log

For the next week, set the intention to capture one unpleasant moment each day. This does not have to be a big deal. It can be something as simple as missing the bus, having to wait in line for coffee, or smiling at someone who didn't smile back. Or it might be bigger, like a fight with a loved one. Again, the closer you can jot down your observations to the time of the event, the better you will likely remember it. But you can also reflect at the end of the day, too; that's fine.

Day	What was the unpleasant event?	What thoughts, feelings, and sensations did you observe during the experience?

Use this space to take notes from today's session—
including the "take-home points."

As part of your between-session practice, you may be asked to listen to one or more audio files. These files may be given to you by your program facilitator, or you can download them from the Treatments That Work website at www. oxfordclinicalpsych.com/WisdomMind.

Congratulations—you have made it to the halfway point in the program! There's a saying, "It takes 28 days to learn a new habit." In the first half of the program, we focus on learning the basic techniques for coming back to the present moment and making them a habit in our lives. This can seem effortful and challenging at times. You can think about mindfulness as "basic hygiene"—most of us wouldn't argue with ourselves about whether we need to brush our teeth or bathe. In the same way, rather than being a chore on our to-do list, mindfulness becomes like basic mental hygiene—we start to feel "icky" if we don't do it!

This week we will also continue making that bridge to daily life with Aimless Wandering, noting your Emotional Weather, and also noticing when you end up "falling down the hole."

Your between-session practices for this week are:

1. (Optional) Read Chapters 18 and 19 from *Full Catastrophe Living* ("Change: The One Thing You Can Be Sure Of" and "Stuck in Stress Reactivity").
2. Do the longer Sitting Practice (Open Monitoring, 40-minute practice) on 3 days. Alternate this with either the Body Scan or one of the Mindful Yoga series for the other 3 days. Fill out the practice log for any time you did any of these three practices.
3. Do the Emotional Weather practice at least 3 days; fill out the corresponding tracking log.
4. Listen to the audio on "Aimless Wandering." Go for an Aimless Wander at least three times during the week, and take note of any observations you make on the corresponding tracking log.
5. Notice when you "fall down the hole" (i.e., reacting versus responding), and take note of this on the corresponding tracking log.

When are you going to practice this week? How will you remember to practice?

My time to practice this week will be:

_____

I will remember to practice by:

_____

_____

For next week: Remember to bring your *Workbook*, a mat/blanket, and your planner/calendar.

Practice Log (Alternating Sitting, Body Scan, and Mindful Yoga)

Please make a note here of what you practiced, when you practiced, and if there were any obstacles to practicing if you did not do it on a particular day.

Day of practice? Which practice did you do?	What did you notice (e.g., thoughts, feelings, sensations)?	What obstacles did you notice getting in the way of doing the practice?

Falling Down the Hole Tracking Log

The poem you just heard is called "Autobiography in Five Chapters," by Portia Nelson. We have already talked about having "slips and falls." Sometimes we can quickly get up again from our falls; other times we end up deep in a hole—sometimes for days, weeks, or even years. The good news is that even if we end up "in the hole," we don't have to be stuck there forever. Mindfulness practice allows us to gain more awareness about where we get stuck in patterns of impulsively **reacting** in the same old ways. Over time, we learn to make choices and respond freshly to the situation. For the next week, start to track where you get stuck in the hole, reacting in old habitual ways. Explore options for **responding** with creativity and openness.

The "hole" where you got stuck	What thoughts, feelings, and sensations did you observe during the experience?

Tracking Log for Emotional Weather, Aimless Wandering, and the Commentator

Emotional Weather: Do this short practice at least three times this week. What did you notice about your experience?

Aimless Wandering: Listen to the audio track that accompanies this practice (5b: Aimless Wandering), and then go for an Aimless Wander. Jot down some reflections about your experience when you return.

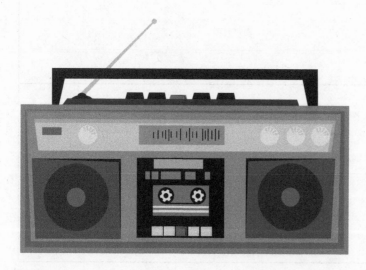

Commentator: Have you ever tried to have a conversation when a radio is playing loudly in the background? It's challenging, isn't it! Our commentator is like that radio—the endless stories and comments make it very hard to pay attention to what is actually happening in our current experience. Continue to notice this week when the commentator takes you away from your experience.

*Use this space to take notes from today's session—
including the "take-home points."*

"It's only with the heart that one sees rightly; what is essential is invisible to the eye."

Antoine de Saint-Exupéry

As part of your between-session practice, you may be asked to listen to one or more audio files. These files may be given to you by your program facilitator, or you can download them from the Treatments That Work website at www. oxfordclinicalpsych.com/WisdomMind.

We are moving toward the end of the program, which means entering some challenging territory. We are continuing to move the practice into our daily life, bringing kindness and curiosity not only to pleasurable experiences but also to those that are more challenging, realizing that sweet and sour both make up the rich, delicious taste of our human life.

Your between-session practices for this week are:

1. (Optional) Read Chapter 20 from *Full Catastrophe Living* ("Responding to Stress Instead of Reacting").
2. Continue to alternate Open Monitoring (long sitting practice) with either the Body Scan or one of the yoga series for 6 days.
3. Read the text provided on communication styles, and notice moments of reacting versus responding in relation to other people.
4. Remember to keep looking for Ordinary Magic (listen to audio track 2a: Ordinary Magic).

When are you going to practice this week? How will you remember to practice?

My time to practice this week will be:

_____

I will remember to practice by:

_____

_____

For next week: Remember to bring your *Workbook*, a mat/blanket, and your planner/calendar.

Practice Log (Alternating Sitting, Body Scan, and Mindful Yoga)

Please make a note here of what you practiced, when you practiced, and if there were any obstacles to practicing if you did not do it on a particular day.

Day of practice? Which practice did you do?	What did you notice (e.g., thoughts, feelings, sensations)?	What obstacles did you notice getting in the way of doing the practice?

Passive, Assertive, and Aggressive Communication Styles

YOUR FEELINGS

Passive	Assertive	Aggressive
You feel anxious, ignored, hurt, manipulated, and disappointed with yourself. You might find yourself feeling angry and resentful later on.	You feel confident and successful. You tend to feel good about yourself at the time and later. You generally feel in control, you have self-respect, and you are goal-oriented.	You feel self-righteous, controlling, and superior. Sometimes you feel embarrassed or selfish later on.

NONVERBAL BEHAVIORS

Passive	Assertive	Aggressive
You use actions instead of words. You hope someone will guess what you want. You look as if you do not mean what you say. Your voice may be weak, hesitant, and soft, speaking in a whisper or monotone. Your eyes may be to the side or downcast. You nod your head to almost anything anyone says. You sit or stand as far away as you can from the other person. You might look uncomfortable, tense, or irritated.	You listen closely. Your manner is calm and assured. You communicate caring and strength. Your voice is firm, yet warm and expressive. You look directly at the other person, facing them, but do not stare. Your hands are relaxed. You hold your head erect and you lean toward the other person. Your expression is relaxed.	You make an exaggerated show of strength. You may come across as flippant or having an air of superiority. Your voice may be tense, loud, or cold, or it may come across as demanding. Your eyes are also narrow and cold. You might take on a fighting stance, with hands on your hips and standing close to the other person. Your hands may be in fists or have fingers pointed toward the other person. You appear tense and angry.

YOUR APPARENT GOALS

Passive	Assertive	Aggressive
To be liked.	To communicate, to be respected.	To dominate or humiliate.

PAYOFFS

<u>Passive</u>	<u>Assertive</u>	<u>Aggressive</u>
You find yourself avoiding unpleasant situations, conflicts, tension, and confrontation. You do not have to take any responsibility for your choices.	You feel quite good. You feel respected by others. Your self-confidence improves. You make your own choices. Your relationships with others are generally good. You have very little physical distress either in the moment or later. You are generally in touch with your feelings.	You manage to get some anger off your chest. You achieve a feeling of control or of being superior.

OTHERS' FEELINGS

<u>Passive</u>	<u>Assertive</u>	<u>Aggressive</u>
In response to your interactions, others might feel guilty, superior, frustrated, or even angry.	In response to your interactions, others tend to feel respected or valued. They feel free to express themselves.	In response to your interactions, others can be left feeling humiliated, unappreciated, or hurt.

OTHERS MAY FEEL FRUSTRATED OR CONFUSED

<u>Passive</u>	<u>Assertive</u>	<u>Aggressive</u>
To be liked.	Others typically respect, trust, and value you. They know where you stand on things.	Others may feel hurt, defensive, humiliated, or angry. They might resent, distrust, and fear you. They may find themselves wanting revenge.

PROBABLE OUTCOME OF EACH TYPE OF BEHAVIOR

<u>Passive</u>	<u>Assertive</u>	<u>Aggressive</u>
You may not get what you want. If you do get your own way, it is in an indirect way. You feel emotionally dishonest. Others achieve their goals at your expense, and as a result, your rights are violated. You might find anger building up and you either suppress it or redirect it to less powerful people. You might procrastinate, suffer in silence, or do things half-heartedly. You might end up feeling lonely or isolated from others.	You often get what you want, so long as it is reasonable. You often achieve your goals. You gain self-respect. You generally feel good. You convert win–lose to win–win. The outcome of situations is determined by above-board negotiations. Everyone's rights—both yours and those of others—are respected at all times.	You might often get what you want, but it comes at the expense of others. You hurt others by making choices on their behalf and infantilizing them. Others may feel a right to "get even" with you. You may find that you have difficulty relaxing and unwinding after interactions. Your relationships ultimately suffer, as fewer people are inclined to engage with you.

Reacting Versus Responding (Mindful Communication)

When we are on auto-pilot, we are unable to make skillful, informed choices. We end up engaging in habitual patterns or having an immediate reaction to the situation. Unfortunately, this more often than not has a negative effect on other people in our life. It might only be after the fact that we actually realize what we have said or done, and by then the moment has passed us by. Mindfulness is about slowing down the speed of our thinking process so that we can see the habitual tendency coming up. Instead of immediately **reacting**, we can make a choice about how to **respond**. We might end up doing something different, or even the same thing, but the point is that it was a choice we made for ourselves. Last week, we talked about getting "stuck in a hole" with ourselves. This week, observe where you get stuck in the hole (react) versus times when you make an informed choice (respond) in your interactions with other people. Pay particular attention to your communication styles.

What was the situation?	Did you react (get stuck) or respond (make a choice)?

Ordinary Magic

This week, remember to bring mindful awareness to routine daily activities, to uncover that "ordinary magic." If helpful, go back and listen to the guided audio that you were introduced to in Session 2 (2a: Ordinary Magic). You might even want to try something completely out of the norm, as an experiment. Maybe there's something you have wanted to try but have been judging or questioning yourself about it. Now is your chance to go for it!

Did You Know?

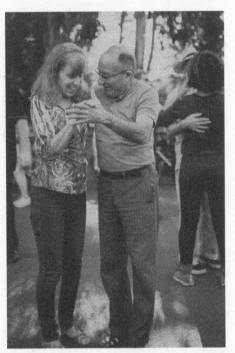

Photo by John Moeses Bauan on Unsplash

In longitudinal studies, researchers have been investigating lifestyle factors that seem to decrease the risk of cognitive decline and eventual Alzheimer's disease. In a recent study, they followed seniors engaged in all kinds of leisure activities, such as swimming, walking, and crossword puzzles. Did you know that the activity that conferred the greatest benefit to seniors was **dancing**? That's right—dancing is both cognitively complex (getting that sequence of steps right!) and physically challenging, as well as providing the inherent enjoyment of good music and laughs with friends. It's also safe to say that the more mindful you are when you do some activity, the more you can "savor the moment" of enjoyment when it occurs. Even if you're too shy to dance in a crowd, find your favorite CD or record, put it on, and just let your body move to the music in a mindful way—let the music move you, instead of you moving the music.

And remember: Dancing and any other leisure activities you enjoy contribute to cognitive reserve—your mental bank account that helps to prevent or slow decline.

*Use this space to take notes from today's session—
including the "take-home points."*

As part of your between-session practice, you may be asked to listen to one or more audio files. These files may be given to you by your program facilitator, or you can download them from the Treatments That Work website at www. oxfordclinicalpsych.com/WisdomMind.

This week, you are encouraged to start thinking about how you will "bring the practice forward" into your life beyond the end of this program. This is what we refer to as *becoming your own meditation instructor*, where you decide what practice you need on a given day. Later in this chapter, details are provided about our upcoming retreat this week, where you will get a taste of an immersion in silent practice.

This week, make the practice your own. Each day, notice where you feel called and follow the call—is it yoga? Or Sitting Practice? Or Aimless Wandering? Trust your own wisdom mind about what needs to happen.

1. Each day, do whatever practice inspires or calls to you.
2. Do the Loving-Kindness practice on at least 3 days.
3. Continue to notice times of reacting versus responding both toward yourself and in relation to other people.
4. Capture bittersweet moments of your life.
5. Think about how you will bring the practice forward when the program is finished.

When are you going to practice this week? How will you remember to practice?

My time to practice this week will be:

_____

I will remember to practice by:

_____

_____

Remember: This weekend we will meet for our 1-day retreat with the entire group of *Wisdom Mind* participants. You are invited to put it in your planner/calendar right now so you don't forget. More information is contained on the following pages about how to prepare for the retreat.

FOR THE PARTICIPANT 7.1

Loving-Kindness Practice (Relating to Our Pain Directly)

"Pain is inevitable; suffering is optional."

Anonymous

Our society is set up in a way that makes it very difficult for us to relate to any kind of pain or discomfort. We receive messages in the media that the only valid way to be in the world is to be always happy and pain-free. We find ourselves endlessly striving for the perfect, comfortable life, the perfect body, and the perfect relationships. Unfortunately, life does not hold very well to that belief system. The reality is that we all experience various types of pain in our lives—we get sick, we lose touch with loved ones, and our dreams and plans may not work out as we thought they would. Pain is just part of the human condition.

Before you start to think this sounds like a hopeless situation . . . wait! While it's true that pain is part of the human experience, suffering is not. Moments of pain come and go, but what makes them feel solid and long-lasting is our resistance to them—that is what causes suffering.

Suffering = Pain × Resistance

Resistance is another word for the commentator, the tendency to judge and reject our painful experience. So how do we begin to work with this? Instead of resisting or rejecting our pain, we can enter into a relationship with it, a conversation to understand what it wants and what it needs. Most of us don't know what the actual pain feels like because we are so wrapped up in the suffering caused by the resistance to it. Earlier, we used the analogy of the commentator as a radio. Through our mindfulness practice, we are able to turn down the volume on that radio, soften our resistance, and relate to the actual experience of pain directly.

This week, you are invited to try the Loving-Kindness Meditation Practice. Listen first to the introductory audio (7a: Loving-Kindness—Introduction), and then follow along with the practice on the separate audio track (7b: Loving-Kindness—Practice Instruction) at least three times. Jot down some notes about what that experience is like.

FOR THE PARTICIPANT 7.2

Reacting Versus Responding

Continue to pay attention to moments where you are reacting as opposed to those where you are responding. When you manage to respond, congratulate yourself for being mindful enough to make that choice. When you find yourself reacting, be kind to yourself (and the other person) and reflect on how you might do things differently next time.

FOR THE PARTICIPANT 7. 3

Handout for Daylong Retreat

This week, we will get to share together an entire day of mindfulness! Sometimes program participants find this prospect quite daunting—that they could take an entire day out of their life for the simple purpose of just being. That said, the vast majority of participants find that being part of the full-day retreat is a unique opportunity to deepen and share their practice with the entire group, and they find that it greatly enhances and solidifies the experience they have accumulated over the course of the program.

How Should You Prepare?

You should bring:

- ✓ Your yoga mat or blanket
- ✓ A cushion to sit on (chairs will also be provided)
- ✓ A "mindful meal"
- ✓ An open mind and heart!

Some other things to know about the retreat:

- Out of respect for your fellow participants, please arrive approximately 5 to 10 minutes early so that you are ready to begin promptly at 9:00 a.m.
- The entire day will be conducted in silence. Please refrain from using your cellphone or checking email during the day. If something emergent comes up, you can take a group facilitator aside to let them know what is happening. But otherwise, it is very important to maintain the "container" of the retreat space for the entire day.
- An important part of the day is a "mindful meal." This offers you a chance to eat together, mindfully, in silence. Try to take time to think of something that would be really worthwhile and delicious for you—good smells, tastes, colors, and so on. The practice begins from the moment you start preparing your meal. Feel free to bring nice silverware, a special glass or cup, and whatever will make the experience special for you.

FOR THE PARTICIPANT 7.4

Bringing the Practice Forward

Learning a new skill in a group can be a very supportive experience for people, a way of sharing the experience and also learning from how other people navigate challenges. Unfortunately, our group must come to an end, and then the real challenge becomes whether we can bring the practice forward, keeping it going after the program has ended. The more we practice mindfulness, the more we can benefit. And just like playing an instrument or dancing or any other skill, we have to use it or lose it. There may be times when we do stop practicing for a while—life's challenges become temporarily overwhelming, and then the practice really is to relate to life directly. But it is important to know that, just like with the breath in Sitting Practice, we can always come back.

Before the last class, reflect on some challenges you can foresee about keeping up the practices after the group is complete. What are some possible solutions to these challenges? Also, reflect on what you have gained from this program and on any new things you have learned about yourself as a result of your participation.

CHAPTER 8

Session 8: Final Session: Taking the Practice Forward

Use this space to take notes from today's session—including the "take-home points."

Three Things You Have Learned About Yourself

It's common along the path of mindfulness to lose our way and stop practicing for a while. The important thing is not to give up completely but, with that beginner's mind, to see it as an opportunity to simply come back. Write down here at least three things you learned about yourself through this practice. Pick things that will motivate you when you have lost your way.

_____

_____

_____

_____

_____

"The Guest House" by Rumi

This being human is a guest house.
Every morning a new arrival.
A joy, a depression, a meanness,
some momentary awareness comes
as an unexpected visitor.
Welcome and entertain them all!
Even if they are a crowd of sorrows,
who violently sweep your house
empty of its furniture,
still, treat each guest honorably.
He may be clearing you out
for some new delight.
The dark thought, the shame, the malice:
Meet them at the door laughing and invite them in.
Be grateful for whatever comes
because each has been sent as a guide from beyond.

Rumi[1]

---

[1] Used with permission from Coleman Barks.

1. Connect with other program participants. Use that connection as a way to provide support and coaching for continued practice. Arrange practice sessions together to discuss and share your practice.

2. Join a formal practice community that uses mindfulness practice. Your facilitator can provide advice and guidance about local mindfulness-based groups in your town or city. While some groups are part of various different Buddhist traditions, you do not have to become a Buddhist to sit with the groups and practice together. Take this as an opportunity to explore, meet new people, and try out different communities. Write down some ideas here:

3. Note that your facilitators may be arranging a "booster session"—ask them whether this applies to you and, if so, when it will be occurring.

Did You Know?

There are many different meditation groups out there, but not all of them follow the philosophy of mindfulness. If it is a different type of practice, you may find it confusing or unhelpful. Mindfulness sometimes goes by the names *shamatha*, *zazen*, or *vipassana*—this might help you in seeking out other groups if you decide to do so on your own.

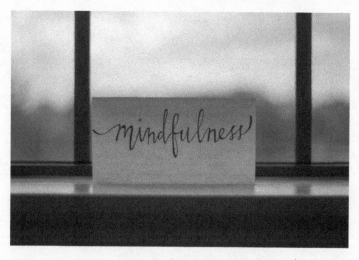

Photo by Lesly Juarez on Unsplash